MW00648936

# ALKALINE DIET COOKBOOK

**Eat Well and Restore Your Health With A 14-Days Meal Plan, Prevent From Degenerative Illness.**

© **Copyright 2019; James Stevenson All rights reserved.**

This document is geared towards providing exact and reliable information with regards to the topic and issue covered. The publication is sold with the idea that the publisher is not required to render accounting, officially permitted, or otherwise, qualified services. If advice is necessary, legal or professional, a practiced individual in the profession should be ordered.

From a Declaration of Principles which was accepted and approved equally by a Committee of the American Bar Association and a Committee of Publishers and Associations.

In no way is it legal to reproduce, duplicate, or transmit any part of this document in either electronic means or in printed format. Recording of this publication is strictly prohibited and any storage of this document is not allowed unless with written permission from the publisher. All rights reserved

The information provided herein is stated to be truthful and consistent, in that any liability, in terms of inattention or otherwise, by any usage or abuse of any policies, processes, or directions contained within is the solitary and utter responsibility of the recipient reader. Under no circumstances will any legal responsibility or blame be held against the publisher for any reparation, damages, or monetary loss due to the information herein, either directly or indirectly.

Respective authors own all copyrights not held by the publisher.

The information herein is offered for informational purposes solely, and is universal as so. The presentation of the information is without contract or any type of guarantee assurance.

The trademarks that are used are without any consent, and the publication of the trademark is without permission or backing by the trademark owner. All trademarks and brands within this book are for clarifying purposes only and are the owned by the owners themselves, not affiliated with this document.

# WHY YOU NEED THIS BOOK

The human body is somewhat alkaline by style. At the point when we expend an extreme measure of corrosive delivering nourishments and not adequate alkaline-framing food sources, we heighten the corrosive body inebriation.

Acidosis will gradually incapacitate our body's crucial functions if we do not quickly take restorative actions. Acidosis, or body over-acidity, remains in truth among the leading causes of human aging. It makes our body extremely susceptible to the series of the fatal degenerative persistent illness, such as diabetes, cancer, arthritis, along with heart diseases.

For this reason, the greatest difficulty we humans have to face to protect our lives is, in fact, to discover properly to lower the production and to optimize the elimination of the body acidic wastes. To prevent acidosis and the age-related diseases, and to continue performing at its greatest level possible, our body requires a healthy lifestyle. This way of life ought to consist of routine exercises, balanced nutrition, a clean physical environment, and a way of living that brings the most affordable stress possible. A healthy way of life permits our body to keep its acid waste material at the lowest level possible.

The alkaline diet, also referred to as the pH wonder diet plan appears to fit the very best of the design of the body. This is primarily due to the fact that it assists in reducing the effects of the acid wastes and permits flushing them out from the body. Individuals should look at alkaline diet as basic dietary boundaries for people to comply with. The individuals who have specific health concerns and special medical diet plans may much better accommodate those diets to alkaline diet boundaries.

# Alkaline Diet Benefits for Diabetics

The great alkaline diet will help upgrade the general soundness of the people experiencing diabetes. As it accomplishes for other people, the alkaline diet will help support their body physiology and digestion, as well as their immune system.

The alkaline diet permits much better management of diabetes and, as an outcome, it helps diabetics prevent more quickly the degenerative diseases connected to their condition. So by following an alkaline diet, in spite of their health circumstance, diabetics can, at the same time, live much healthier and extend their life expectancy significantly.

Diabetics Acid-Alkaline Food Chart

In general, individuals who wish to follow an alkaline diet require to pick their daily food products from an 'Acid-Alkaline Foods Chart.' We just recently released a 'Diabetics Acid-Alkaline Food Chart.' Making use of this particular chart allows diabetics to conform to both the alkaline diet rule and the glycemic index rule.

The alkaline diet rule sets basic dietary guidelines. According to this diet strategy, our everyday food intake should be composed of a minimum of 80 percent of alkaline-forming foods, and of no more than 20 percent of acidifying foodstuff. Additionally, the diet plan highlights that the more alkaline a food item is, the much better it is actually; and on the other hand, the more acidifying a food is, the even worse it ought to be for the body.

Concerning the glycemic list rule, it isolates nourishments into four primary arrangements as to their ability to raise the glucose level. This capacity is presently estimated by the glycemic file GI that extents from 0 to 100. Foods that consist of almost no carbs which have, in effect, a negligible glycemic index (GI ~ 0); diabetics might take them easily. Foods including carbs with a low glycemic index (GI 55 or less); people with diabetes must eat these products with some safety measure. Foods that have carbs of the high glycemic index (GI 56 or more); diabetics must, up until now as possible, exclude them from their diet. Processed foods; diabetics will require to speak with the manufacturers' labels to find out their specific glycemic index values.

# Contents

# INTRODUCTION

The alkaline diet is also understood as the acid-alkaline diet plan or the alkaline ash diet. It is based around the idea that the foods you consume leave behind an "ash" residue after they have been metabolized. This ash can be acid or alkaline.

Proponents of this diet plan claim that certain foods can impact the level of acidity and alkalinity of physical fluids, consisting of urine and blood. If you consume foods with acidic ash, they make the body acidic They make the body alkaline if you eat foods with alkaline ash.

Acid ash is thought to make you susceptible to illness such as muscle, osteoporosis, and cancer wasting, whereas alkaline ash is considered to be protective. To ensure you remain alkaline, it is advised that you keep an eye on your urine, utilizing helpful pH test strips.

For those who do not completely comprehend human physiology and are not nutrition specialists, diet claims like this sound rather convincing. However, is it actually real? The following will unmask this myth and clear up some confusion relating to the alkaline diet plan.

However, first, it is needed to comprehend the meaning of the pH value.

Put just; the pH value is a measure of how acidic or alkaline something is. The pH worth ranges from 0 to 14.

0-7 is acidic.

7 is neutral

7-14 is alkaline

For instance, the stomach is filled with extremely acidic hydrochloric acid, a pH value between 2 and 3.5. The level of acidity assists in eliminating germs and break down food.

On the other hand, human blood is constantly a little alkaline, with a pH of between 7.35 to 7.45. Usually, the body has a number of reliable systems (gone over later) to keep the blood pH within this range. Falling out of it is really severe and can be fatal.

# Results Of Foods On Urine And Blood pH

Foods leave an acid or alkaline ash. Acid ash consists of phosphate and sulfur. Alkaline ash includes calcium, magnesium, and potassium.

Certain food groups are thought about acidic, neutral, or alkaline.
Acidic: Meats, fish, dairy, eggs, grains, and alcohol.
Neutral: Fats, starches, and sugars.
Alkaline: Fruits, nuts, vegetables, and veggies.

## Urine pH

Foods you consume change the pH of your urine. If you have a green smoothie for breakfast, your urine, in a couple of hours, will be more alkaline than if you had bacon and eggs.
For somebody on an alkaline diet plan, urine pH can be extremely quickly monitored and may even supply instantaneous satisfaction. Urine pH is neither a good sign of the overall pH of the body, nor is it a great indicator of general health.

## Blood pH.

Foods you eat do not alter your blood pH. When you eat something with acid ash like protein, the acids produced are rapidly neutralized by bicarbonate ions in the blood. This reaction produces carbon dioxide, which is breathed out through the lungs, and salts, which are excreted by the kidneys in your urine.

During the procedure of excretion, the kidneys produce brand-new bicarbonate ions, which are returned to the blood to change the bicarbonate that was initially used to neutralize the acid. This makes a maintainable cycle where the body can save the pH of the blood inside a tight assortment.

As long as your kidneys are working typically, your blood pH will not be affected by the foods you consume, whether they are acidic or alkaline. The claim that consuming alkaline foods will make your body or blood pH more alkaline is not true.

## Acidic Diet And Cancer

Those who advocate an alkaline diet plan claim that it can treat cancer because cancer can just grow in an acidic environment. By consuming an alkaline diet, cancer cells can not die but grow.

Cancer grows in regular body tissue, which has a somewhat alkaline pH of 7.4. Lots of experiments have validated this by successfully growing cancer cells in an alkaline environment.

Nevertheless, cancer cells do grow faster with the level of acidity. As soon as growth starts to develop, it develops its own acidic environment by breaking down glucose and minimizing blood circulation. Therefore, it is not the acidic environment that triggers cancer; however, cancer that triggers the acidic environment.

A lot more intriguing is a 2005 research study by the National Cancer Institute which uses vitamin C (ascorbic acid) to deal with cancer. They found that by administering pharmacologic doses intravenously, ascorbic acid successfully eliminated cancer cells without damaging typical cells. This is another case of disease cells being powerless against causticity, rather than alkalinity.

Simply put, there is no clinical link between eating an acidic diet and cancer. Cancer cells can grow in both acidic and alkaline environments.

## Acidic Diet And Osteoporosis

Osteoporosis is a progressive bone disease defined by a reduction in bone mineral material, causing lowered bone density and strength and greater danger of a broken bone.

Proponents of the alkaline diet think that in order to maintain a consistent blood pH, the body takes alkaline minerals like calcium from the bones to reduce the effects of the acids from an acidic diet plan. As gone over above, this is definitely not real. The kidneys and the respiratory system are responsible for regulating blood pH, not the bones.

Many research studies have actually shown that increasing animal protein intake is favorable for bone metabolism as it increases calcium retention and activates IGF-1 (insulin-like development factor-1) that stimulates bone regeneration. Therefore, the hypothesis that an acidic diet plan triggers bone loss is not supported by science.

## Acidic Diet And Muscle Wasting

Supporters of the alkaline diet think that in order to get rid of excess acid brought on by an acidic diet, the kidneys will steal amino acids (building blocks of protein) from muscle tissues, causing muscle loss. The proposed mechanism resembles the one causing osteoporosis.

As discussed, blood pH is controlled by the kidneys and the lungs, not the muscles. Hence, acidic foods like meats, dairy, and eggs do not cause muscle loss. As a matter of truth, they are total dietary proteins that will support muscle repair work and assistance avoid muscle wasting.

# WHAT DID OUR ANCESTORS EAT?

A variety of research studies have actually analyzed whether our pre-agricultural forefathers ate net acidic or net alkaline diets. Extremely surprisingly, they found that about half of the hunter-gatherers consumed net acid-forming diets, while the other half consumed net alkaline-forming diets.

Acid-forming diet plans were more typical as people moved even more north of the equator — the less hospitable the environment, the more animal proteins they consumed. In more tropical environments where vegetables and fruits were abundant, their diet ended up being more alkaline.

From an evolutionary viewpoint, the theory that acidic or protein-rich diets trigger illnesses like cancer, muscle, and osteoporosis loss is not legitimate. Half of the hunter-gatherers were consuming net acid-forming diet plans, yet, they had no evidence of such degenerative illness.

It deserves noting that there is no one-size-fits-all diet plan that works for everyone, which is why Metabolic Typing is so practical in determining your optimum diet. Due to our genetic differences, some individuals will gain from an acidic diet plan, some an alkaline diet plan, and some in between. Thus the saying: one guy's food can be another man's poison.

## Final Thoughts

It is true that lots of people who have changed to an alkaline diet plan see considerable health improvements. Do bear in mind that other factors may be at work:

If you change to an alkaline diet, you are immediately consuming more veggies and fruits. When you consume more vegetables and fruits, you are most likely eating less processed foods too.

Consuming less dairy and eggs will benefit those who are lactose-intolerant or have a food sensitivity to eggs, which is rather common among the basic population.

Consuming fewer grains will benefit those who are gluten-sensitive or have a dripping gut or autoimmune illness.

## Alkaline Water

Anyways, it is not real. Water that is too alkaline can be detrimental to your health and lead to dietary disequilibrium.

If you consume alkaline water all the time, it will neutralize your stomach acid and raise the alkalinity of your stomach. Over time, it will impair your ability to absorb food and absorb nutrients and minerals. With less acidity in the stomach, it will also unlock for germs and parasites to enter into your small intestine.

The bottom line is that alkaline water is not the answer to great health. Tidy, filtered water is still the finest water for your                                                          body.

# THE ALKALINE DIET: A LITTLE-KNOWN AND POWERFUL WEIGHT LOSS PLAN

What if you knew about a weight loss program that would help you lose weight and feel younger? Would you try it? The alkaline diet and way of life have actually been around for over 60 years, yet lots of people aren't familiar with its natural, safe and tested weight loss properties!

The alkaline diet plan is not a gimmick or a fad. It's a healthy and easy way to take pleasure in brand-new levels of health. In this section, you'll learn about what this dietary strategy is, what makes it different, and how it can produce life-changing results for you, your waistline and your health.

Are you enjoying a sexy and slim body today? If so, you're in the minority.

Sadly, over 65 percent of Americans are either overweight or overweight. If you're obese, you probably experience signs of ill-health like tiredness, swelling, sore joints, and a host of other signs of poor health.

Even worse yet, you most likely feel like quitting on ever delighting in the body you want and are worthy of. Maybe you've been informed that you're simply growing older, but that just isn't the reality. Don't purchase into that lie. Other cultures have healthy, lean elders who take pleasure in excellent health into their nineties!

The reality is, your body is a brilliantly created device and if you have any symptoms of ill-health, this is a sure sign that your body's chemistry is too acidic. This is since the body does not simply break down one day.

# WHAT'S INCORRECT WITH THE WAY YOU'RE CONSUMING NOW?

The Standard American Diet (S.A.D.) focuses on fine-tuned carbs, sugars, alcohol, meats, and dairy. These foods are all extremely acid-forming. In spite of pleas from the nutritional experts, we simply do not eat enough of the alkalizing foods such as fresh fruits, veggies, beans, and nuts.

In short, our S.A.D. way of life upsets the natural acid-alkaline balance our bodies require. This condition triggers weight problems, low-level pains and discomforts, colds and influenza, and eventually illness sets in.

We've lost our way. This is where an alkaline diet can assist in restoring our health.

I'm sure you're familiar with the term pH, which describes the level of acidity or alkalinity that consisted of something. Alkalinity is determined on a scale. You can take an economical and simple test in your home to see where your alkalinity level falls, as well as to monitor it frequently.

Medical researchers and scientists have understood for at least 70 years this lesser-known fact ... your body needs a certain pH level, or the delicate balance of your body's acid-alkaline levels - for optimal health and vitality.

You may believe ..." I don't need to know all this chemistry. What does the appropriate pH balance and alkalinity matter to me?" I understand these were my questions when I first found out about alkaline consuming.

We'll utilize two examples of how acid and alkalinity contributes to your body.

We all understand that our stomach has acid in it. Along with enzymes, this acid is necessary for breaking food into standard components that can be absorbed by the digestive system. We would pass away from malnutrition in no time because the body could not utilize a whole piece of meat or an entire piece of anything, for that matter!

2: Different parts of our body require various levels of acidity or alkalinity. Your blood requires a slightly more alkaline level than your stomach acids.

While these examples show that the numerous parts or systems in the body require different pH levels, we don't need to fret about that.

ur problem is basic and it's this ... we are simply to acidic overall, period. , if you're interested in discovering more about pH, you can discover tons of info on the web by just searching the term.

The essential thing to know is this. When your body is too acidic over a very long time, it causes numerous illnesses like weight problems, arthritis, bone density loss, high blood pressure, heart problem and stroke. The list is limitless since the body just quits the battle for vitality and goes into survival mode as long as it can.

# AN ALKALINE DIET PLAN IS UNIQUE

Many diet plans concentrate on the same foods that cause you to be ill or obese in the first location. They just ask you to eat less of those things, to consume more time each day, or to integrate them differently.

In fairness to these diet plan's creators, they know that many of us do not desire to make the larger modifications for our health. We like a diet that's concentrated on processed and fine-tuned foods, our meat, our sugar, alcohols, and such. The diet developers are simply attempting to help us make easier changes.

We've gotten utilized to eating by doing this, and it's not ALL our fault! Greedy food processing giants have a vested interest in keeping us eating this method. Earnings are much higher in this sector of the food market than in the production of your more standard foods like fruits and veggies.

So, once again, YES ... this diet plan is various. Healthy and important, you would not require to read this short article. If those other diets worked, you would you would be feeling lean. You wouldn't need a dietary change.

Here's a partial list of foods that you can eat freely in an alkaline diet:

- Fresh fruits and freshly made juices
- Fresh veggies and juices
- Cooked veggies
- Some vegetables and soy
- Lean proteins and some eggs
- Specific grains
- Healthy fats and nuts

You might be shocked to discover that some veggies and fruits are better for you than others!

You can take in minimal quantities of these foods and beverages:
- Dairy
- Lots of typical grains
- Refined foods and sugars
- Alcohol and caffeine


What's it like to be on the alkaline diet plan, and what results can you anticipate?

Like any modification in diet or way of life, you'll go through an adjustment duration. Yet since you're burning the cleanest fuel, which your body craves, so unlike numerous diet plan plans, you will not ever need to feel starving. Plus, you can eat all you like up until you're pleased. You likewise won't need to count calories. And you'll enjoy a lot of variety, so you'll never ever get tired of eating.

Consider an alkaline diet as a kind of 'juice fast' for the body. Only it's not so severe. You're consuming nutrient-dense, easily digestible foods that your body longs for. When you provide all the cells of the body that it so frantically requires, your hunger disappears. And there's no need to stress over uninteresting veggies since there are lots of tasty dishes found on the internet and in books.


With all the diet plans there, why should you think about an alternative strategy like the alkaline diet?

Many reviews exist where individuals report losing over two pounds each week. Plus your skin will end up being more flexible once again, your energy will increase, and you'll feel younger.

Plus, the alkaline diet does two crucial things that traditional diet plans do not.
1. It supplies remarkable nourishment to your body's cells.
2. It naturally assists to cleanse and cleanse the cells, too.

These two truths lag the reason why an alkaline diet works so quickly and safely.

When considering an alkaline diet. Given that it's can be rather various from the method you might be used to consuming, you might question if you can go back to your former eating habits. When you have lost all your weight, the sincere answer is that it's clever to continue as many of the concepts as you can. It doesn't need to be all or nothing. Anything you do to embrace a much healthier diet plan will greatly increase your chances of keeping the weight off for good.

# BACK TO BASICS WITH AN ALKALINE DIET

When you pick to eat an alkaline diet, you are really eating foods that are really comparable to what man was created to consume. If you take a look at what our forefathers ate, you will find a diet abundant in fresh fruits, veggies, beans, nuts, and fish. Man's diet plan today is often complete of foods that are high in unhealthy fats, salt, cholesterol, and acidifying foods.

## How Our Diet Changed

Some individuals think that man's diet changed just recently, the shift from a mainly alkaline diet plan to an acid diet in fact began thousands of years ago. Our original diet plan consisted of foraged fruits, veggies and nuts, along with whatever meat could be captured. The end outcome was a diet plan that was still much healthier than what many people consume today; however the shift from alkaline to acid had begun.

## Recent Dietary Changes

It's obvious that our contemporary diet plan consists of numerous foods that are not healthy for us. Excessive unhealthy food and "quick food" has actually decreased the quality of our diet. Obesity has actually ended up being the standard and, in addition to it, a higher incidence of illness such as diabetes, coronary disease, and cancer. If you wish to enhance your health and minimize the risk of numerous illnesses, an alkaline diet plan can assist get your body back to basics.

## What is an Alkaline Diet?

They produce either an alkalizing or acidifying impact within the body when foods are eaten and digested. Some individuals get confused because the real pH of the food itself does not have anything to do with the impact of the food as soon as it is digested. At the point when increasingly alkaline nourishments are devoured, the body can turn out to be marginally alkaline rather than corrosive.Preferably, the blood pH level needs to be between 7.35 and 7.45. Foods such as citrus fruits, soy items, raw vegetables and fruits, wild rice, almonds, and natural sweeteners such as Stevia are all excellent alkaline food options.

## Advantages of an Alkaline Diet

It's much easier to lose weight or preserve a healthy weight level on an alkaline diet plan. Allergic reactions are frequently eased as an outcome of an alkaline diet plan. The majority of people find that they just feel much better, with an increased sense of health and well-being, once they make a conscious effort to adhere to an alkaline diet.

# ALKALINE DIET GUIDELINES

In this chapter, we will be going over the alkaline diet plan standards. Initially, we should discover the alkaline diet. The alkaline diet plan is likewise known as the ph miracle, ph balance diet, or the acid alkaline diet plan, to name a few things. It based on the theory that whatever you consume can either trigger your body to develop up acid or to end up being more alkaline. For someone beginning this diet, it can be frustrating attempting to find out what is great (alkaline) and what is bad( acidic). This is why I have actually decided to create the alkaline diet standards and so clear up a few of the confusion.

There are lots of alkaline diet plan standards. The standard concept is specific compounds are worse for the body then others. One of the alkaline diet plan guidelines is that you should try to eat 75-80% alkaline. It is indicating that 75-80% of your diet plan is from the alkaline food chart. Certain foods are thought about more acid forming than others. To give you an idea here is a list of foods that are thought about highly acid forming according to the alkaline diet standards: sweeteners (equal, low and sweet, nutra-sweet, and aspartame among others) beer, salt, jam, ice cream, beef, lobster, fried food, processed cheese, and soft beverages. Here is a fun truth soda has a ph of 2.5. This is highly acidic. In order to reduce the effects of on can of cola, you would need to drink 32 glasses of water.

On the other side of the spectrum, there isa particular food that are thought about to by highly alkaline and when ingested, helps increases the alkalinity of the body. According to the alkaline diet plan standards, these food are as follows: sea salt, lotus rood, watermelon, tangerines, sweet potato, lime, pineapple, seaweed, pumpkin seeds, and lentils.

The alkaline diet plan guidelines state that drugs are exceptionally acid forming as well. Think of all those individuals who take some type of drug to reduce their heartburn. Bit do they understand their short-lived solution is causing bigger problems for them in the long run. There are many other alkaline diet foods; this was simply an example. The more you eat the much better you will feel. Often times, individuals experience a period of detoxing when they change to the alkaline diet plan. The alkaline diet standards suggest that you got through a period of a couple of weeks in detox to rid your body of toxic substances and enable to adapt to this entirely brand-new way of consuming

.

# CHOOSING ALKALINE DIETS IS THE ONLY WAY TO LIVE A HEALTHY LIFESTYLE

The low carbohydrate and high protein diets doing the rounds these days are an invitation to bad health. If an in shape body is to be kept, one needs to guide completely clear of such diets; all athletes know that. Not just do they result in severe tiredness but also are a disaster where weight management is concerned. Selecting alkaline diet plans is the only method to live a healthy life as well as shed those additional pounds.

Alkaline diets require one to follow a life design entirely opposite of the high protein low carbohydrate diet plans. The high protein diet plans leave the person following it, fatigued and tired. It is for those who lead a stagnant life and wish to shed some weight. However, the weight that is lost comes back on as soon as one stops the diet. With alkaline diets this isn't the situation. The diet plans can be coordinated into ones way of life and inside days the outcomes start to show.They need one to expend around 80 % alkalizing nourishments to keep the alkaline ph of the body to 7.4. High protein diets will, in general, make the ph of the body acidic rather than its regular alkaline tilt. At the point when the body ph winds up being acidic, it attracts all sicknesses and exhausts one of vitality. An acidic ph likewise brings about quick degeneration of the human body cells. That leads to reduced life. One needs to stay away from these crash diets and take a look at achieving health and vitality by following alkaline diets instead.

Alkaline diet plans lead to the body ph preserving its alkaline nature. The various body functions are brought out smoothly and the immune system of the body stays strong. In other words, they assist drive away diseases as opposed to high protein diets that appear to attract them.

Alkaline diet plans constitute primarily of fruits and vegetables. One ought to try and consume green veggies and sweet fruits so that they comprise about 70 to 80 percent of their overall food consumption. Melons and lemons should likewise be eaten. Almonds, honey, and olive oil are likewise high on the list of foods to be taken in for following alkaline diets. Fats and meats must be prevented. All nourishments that are acidifying like espresso, liquor, meats, and even specific veggies like cooked spinach needs not to shape over 20% of ones diet. Alkaline water is also a should for everyone desiring to improve their diet. At least 6 to 8 glasses of alkaline water can do wonders for your body cleaning. Processed food is all likewise high and acidic on weight getting compounds; therefore,it needs to be prevented. Drinks like sodas are extremely acidic and ought to not be consumed at all. It takes 32 glasses of water to cancel one glass of soda.

Alkaline diets are for everyone. Each one of us ought to stop abusing our bodies and look at a healthy and long life by making alkaline diets a part of our lifestyle.

# ACID ALKALINE DIET BENEFITS & WHY IT IS RECOMMENDED

In the event that you have known about the Atkins diet, at that point, the Acid Alkaline Diet is the all out switch of that. The Atkins diet plan is a high protein, high fat however low carbs diet. An Acid alkaline, likewise understood as an alkaline ash diet plan, alkaline acid diet and the alkaline diet, keeps the ph level of the body well balanced and so safeguards against different health problems.

The basis of a diet plan that is acid alkaline lies in the fact that our body ph preferably needs to be a 7.3.This somewhat alkaline degree of the body ph keeps all the essential organs working great, just as the retention of various minerals is upgraded. At the point when this ph tilts to the acidic side difficulty begins creating. An acidic ph level prompts practically all body parts enduring in one strategy or the other. Presently since our body should be alkaline in nature it must reflect in our nourishment utilization as well. Foods that are alkalizing need to be taken in mush more as opposed to the acidifying foods. Equated in a simpler language, this would imply more of vegetable and fruit intake and very low meats and oil consumption. , if the body's alkaline minerals such as magnesium, calcium and potassium levels drop so will its health causing it to degenerate and its defenses to drop guard. An alkaline diet protects that from occurring. A corrosive alkaline or an alkaline debris diet plan comprises of 80% alkalizing nourishments and 20 % acidic nourishments. Because the alkaline acid ratio in the body needs to be one is to 4 our food intake should be of comparable nature.

Pressure and a low vitality level should both be possible away with a diet that is corrosive alkaline. The individuals who experience the ill effects of incessant viral fevers or the individuals who have a nasal blockage a considerable lot of the time can have more advantageous existences in the event that they have a diet that is corrosive alkaline.

A more prominent degree of vegetable admission is proposed in an alkaline debris diet plan. Lemons must be crushed into water drinks. Millet or quinoa is favored over wheat, olive oil over oil and soups like miso are extremely advantageous for following an alkaline debris diet plan.

If an acid alkaline diet is followed, lost health and vitality can be restored, and lots of chronic diseases prevented as well as treated. It is a fairly simple diet plan, which ought to adjust for a longer and much healthier life span.

# ACID TO ALKALINE DIET, HOW TO LOSE WEIGHT AND LIVE A HEALTHIER LIFESTYLE NATURALLY

The acid to alkaline diet is ending up being a more talked about subject nowadays; however, still, most of the population is uninformed of what it is. Individuals who pass away young, have health issues, struggle with weight problems and so on, usually have an extremely acidic internal environment whereas individuals who live to very old age and don't experience major illness have an internal environment that is more alkaline in nature.

In the modern Western world, the large bulk of people live an extremely unhealthy way of life, predominantly consuming junk and unhealthy food and being constantly exposed to other elements that considerably impact our health in an unfavorable method, in drastic contrast to the acid to an alkaline diet plan. According to the World Health Organization (WHO), there are more that a person billion obese grownups world-wide, with around 300 million of them medically obese. This fact is frightening and is significantly increasing daily!

As a healthcare professional myself, people frequently ask me what the finest ways to stay healthy are. I often tell my clients that in order for us to live a healthy life, not be over weight, avoid serious diseases and diseases and generally live to excellent aging with vigor and vigour, it is important that we take note of the acid to an alkaline diet plan. By observing your bodies pH levels and eating appropriately to ensure your body is more alkaline than acidic, people experience things like quick weight-loss (by a sped up fat disposal procedure), they will live longer, feel less stressed, have a better immune system, improve and more relaxing sleep, have more energy and can likewise experience an increase in libido. These advantages alone are obviously of significant significance to health, durability and happy life. By enabling the body to detox in this way through the acid to alkaline diet people also have actually an increased ability to absorb vitamins and minerals and help prevent many nasty illnesses including cancer and arthritis. With a more alkaline body, stress and pressure on the internal organs arealleviated, skin, bones and cells help and regenerate keep you younger.

Conversely, if an individual's body is too acidic they can easily experience weight problems by holding and gaining onto fat, they will age quicker, a lack of energy will be common, they will quickly and regularly bring in illness and virus' and create an internal environment where yeast and germs can easily thrive.

The majority of people living in the Western world do not follow an acid to alkaline diet plan and are normally more on the acidic scale. This is due mostly to our diet. Some other surprises that likewise trigger acidic construct up include rice, tuna, oats and cheese, so these foods are to be restricted when following an acid to an alkaline diet plan.

Optimum pH to get all the advantages from alkalinity is 7.4 pH. If your body goes 3-4 points, in any case, you will pass away! The pH scale is as follows:

- 0 = total acid/battery acid, hydrochloric acid
- 1 = stomach juices
- 2 = vinegar
- 3 = beer
- 4 = red wine, tomato juice
- 5 = rain
- 6 = milk
- 7 = distilled water
- 8 = sea water
- 9 = baking soda
- 10 = cleaning agent, milk of magnesia
- 11 = ammonia, lime water
- 12 = bleach
- 13 = lye
- 14 = Total Alkaline/Sodium Hydroxide

The acid to an alkaline diet will help your body remain at the optimal variety, around 7.4 pH. The body's reaction to attempting to keep this acid, alkaline balance, is both remarkable and amazing. When your body is too acidic, it attempts whatever to get to a more alkaline state. When this occurs the body shops some acid in your fat to keep it from doing damage to our body which is an advantage, but your body then holds on to the fat for defense, causing the person to gain weight.

When there is excess acid internally, the body discovers alkaline elsewhere from your bones and teeth but your bones and teeth get such drained pipes that they become frail and begin to decay. This can lead to lots of illnesses of the bones and teeth including arthritis and dental caries. If a person were following an acid to an alkaline diet, this would not happen.

The construct up of acid normally will settle far from your much healthier organs but instead, it gravitates towards your weakest organs that are already susceptible to illness. It's like a pack of wolves searching for the weakest among the herd, choosing off the simple victim. As your weaker organs are targeted, it makes it a lot easier for major diseases to embed in, consisting of cancer. It is very important to understand that cancer cells end up being dormant if you are at 7.4 pH (which is the body's optimal pH levels), therefore additional highlighting the significance of maintaining a healthy pH level in our bodies by following the acid to an alkaline diet plan.

When there is an acid in the system, it also contaminates your blood stream. This, in turn, prevents the blood's ability to deliver oxygen to the tissues. RBC's are surrounded by an unfavorable charge so they can bounce off each other and move around in the blood extremely rapidly and deliver their goodness.

In any case, when you are too acidic they lose their negative charge and they stick, triggering them to move extremely gradually. This causes them to struggle to provide nutrients and oxygen in our system. Among the first symptoms of this poisoning is you begin to feel a loss of energy even though you are getting sufficient sleep. Starting an acid to an alkaline diet can fix this really quickly. Your blood likewise has this reaction after drinking alcohol.

Let's put all this into perspective; it takes about 33 glasses of water to neutralize one glass of coke! I'm not even going to mention here what it requires to neutralize a few of the other things that we are taking into our bodies; I believe you understand!

One terrific method to regularly make your body more alkaline is by having green beverages daily. They are very easy to make, taste fantastic and are loaded with vitamins, minerals and chlorophyll which fuel our body. Chlorophyll is a huge part of the acid to an alkaline diet and is the green blood of plants. It is an extremely powerful detoxify-er, blood contractor, cleaner and oxygen booster. The benefits of chlorophyll on our bodies are far too many to include in this book.

# ALKALINE DIET - WHAT YOU SHOULD KNOW ABOUT ITS HEALTH BENEFITS

The food that we take today is totally various from our forefathers and is completely different from what we are so accustomed to these days. A view at the grocery store will shock you with aisles and aisles of processed food items and animal products.

Fad diets are being partly to blame for presenting entire new eating habits, this includes high-protein diets. Recently, usage of animal items and refined food products has actually increased as increasingly more people exclude the day-to-day supply of vegetables and fruits in their diet plans.

Some health specialists connect these diseases to the type of foods we eat. There are particular types of food that interfere with the balance in our body that, throughout such instances, health issues occur.

## Why Alkaline Is Important For Our Body

For a healthy body, the alkaline and acid ration needs to be balanced, which is determined by the pH level in the body. pHworths vary from 0 to 14 and 7 is thought about neutral. Any value less than 7 is thought about acidic. Fine-tuned food, such as meat and meat derivatives, sweets, and some sweetened drinks usually produce a terrific amount of acid for the body.

Acidosis, a case of the high level of acidic in the blood stream and body cells is the common index for the various currentillness inflicting many individuals. Some health specialists conclude that acidosis is accountable for the critical illness suffered by numerous people nowadays.

Alkaline or alkaline diet plans, which generally present in our body, neutralize the high level of acidic in the body to accomplish a balanced state. This is the primary function of the alkaline in the body. However, the presence of the alkaline in the body is rapidly depleted due to the high level of acidic contents it has to reduce the effects of and there is inadequate alkaline food taken in to renew the loss alkaline.

## A Balance Alkaline-Acid Level For A Healthy Body

As explained formerly, acidosis triggers many health-related problems. An important level of acid enter our system, breaking the cells and organs when not neutralize correctly. To prevent this, one needs to see to it that a balanced pH is preserved.

To check whether our body consists of a greater level of alkaline can be carried out with ease — this with using pH strips that are available from any pharmacy. There are two kinds of strips, one for the saliva and the other for urine.

Normally, a saliva pH level strip will determine the level of acid your body is producing; the regular worths must be between 6.5 and 7.5 throughout the day. A urine pH level strip will reveal the level of acid; a regular reading needs to be between 6.0 and 6.5 in the morning and in between 6.5 and 7.0 during the night

High Level of Acidity Is Harmful to the Body

If you consistently experience tiredness, headaches and having regular acute rhinitis and flu, these signs show a high level of acid in the body. The effect of acidosis in the body not only inhibits the typical diseases that we understand; however, other diseases that you might suffer are triggered by a high level of acid in the body.

Anxiety, high acidity, ulcer, dry skin, acne and overweight are a few of those linked with a severe level of acidity in our body. Not limited to these, other crucial and severe illnesses such as joint diseases, osteoporosis, bronchitis, frequent infections and heart problem.

Even with medications, the symptoms might be disguised and continue to impact your health as the root of the issue has actually not been totally gotten rid of. Taking more medication will just intensify the issue as the anti-inflammatory medicine will include the acidic level in the body.

## Alkaline Diet - A Sure Bet To A Healthy Body

In order to reach the root of the diseases, our systems pH value must be maintained in a healthy state. Naturally taking place, alkaline foods have the ability to supplement the lost alkaline levels in the body throughout reducing the effects of the procedure. By keeping a healthy alkaline diet plan, a sufficient amount of alkaline is replenished in the system, therefore, bringing the body back to the predominant alkaline state.

The very basic very first action is to reduce the amount of refined food intake. As we currently know, these foods consist of lots of chemicals, which are the perpetrators in increasing the acidic level in our body.

Oranges and lemons known for being acidic convert into alkaline after food digestion and taken in by the body is a great alkaline diet. Generally, we must take in 75% of alkaline food daily. The greater the number of alkaline foods we took into our system, the higher the neutralization of the acidic condition in our body.

# WHAT IS AN ACID ALKALINE DIET?

A lot of individuals have been struggling to discover the very best diet plan program suitable for them. One of the most common misstatements that these people have is their desire to slim down. They fail to put the essential focus on how to be healthy. If you would like to know the very best diet plan that is perfect for you, then you better ensure it's healthy and is not destroying your body.

## The Alkaline Diet

What is an alkaline diet plan and is this diet healthy for you? This diet plan all started when experts attempted thinking about the pH level of the body. Once the pH level is high, then the environment is alkaline.

This diet is essentially all about eating foods that can promote an alkaline environment in the body while not consuming foods that promote acidity to the body. To start off, foods that can promote an alkaline environment in the body are considered healthy.

The other principle of an alkaline diet plan is to prevent acid foods because these are foods that can make your body at risk for weight gain, heart issues, kidney and liver illness. Few of the numerous acid foods consist of caffeine, foods with high preservatives like canned goods, sodas, fish, meat, alcohol and foods with high sugar material. When you concern think of it, the alkaline diet is not uncommon for everybody, specifically when discussing a healthy diet plan.

## Real Deal with Alkaline Diet

According to specialists, acidic foods can reduce the pH of an individual's urine. When the pH is abnormally low kidney stones tend to form. To counteract this circumstance, an individual requires to increase the pH through consuming alkaline rich foods, that simple.

Given that an alkaline diet plan means preventing alcohol and any other foods with high acidity, it also suggests that you will decrease the threat of developing diseases connected with unhealthy diet plans like diabetes, high blood pressure, and obesity. No precise evidence can prove; some researchers have mentioned that the alkaline diet plan can minimize the danger of cancer.

## Things to Remember

In order for the alkaline diet to work, you should condition yourself to stick to the diet program. Then you much better do it when it requires you to prevent unhealthy foods and beverages. Water treatment is an excellent alternative drink for soda and alcohol. In addition, so that you will not have a tough time finding out which are alkaline and which are acid foods, it is finest that you make a list of each category. Possibly you can look into online on what foods are rich in alkaline and those having high acid material. Because the bulk of foods belong to vegetables and fruits classification, alkaline foods are not that hard to point

.

# WHY THE ALKALINE DIET AND CANCER IS AN IDEAL SOLUTION

As an outcome of the epidemic of cancer that has actually broken out recently, there have actually been fantastic strides made in where cancer came from, how it grows in the body and how reliable alkaline diet plan and cancer program has actually become. The definition of cancer permits the client to have some control in the avoidance and fight of cancer cells. By adhering to a mainly alkaline diet, this lowers, and in fact, satiates, the production of cancer, and other illnesses. Since of this, an alkaline diet has actually been discovered to prevent illness, while an acidic diet plan encourages disease and cancer to grow.

When you take the meaning of cancer merely, it is 'a malformed cell.' This malformed cell can only reproduce malformed cells, and given that the body replicates tens of thousands of cells daily, the answer is to stop that recreation. The very best defense then is a good offense, which is what an alkaline diet does as it feeds the good cells while choking out the illness.

The foods that are taken into the body normally originate from two classifications - foods that produce an acidic environment and foods that produce an alkaline environment. If you are taking a large number of medications, this may cause your system to lean more towards the acidic. However, it can be combated by taking in more alkaline-producing foods.

An alkaline diet is normally made up of alkaline-producing foods so that the pH level is given a level of around 7.4. , if you browse online, there are alkaline/acidic charts of all the foods. Make a copy of the chart and carry it with you when you go or shop out to consume if you are just beginning this diet. In basic, stay away from processed foods, junk foods fried in trans fat, any food made with white sugar or white flour, and all foods with chemicals and steroids. These foods all feed cancer cells. If this is what your diet is comprised of, examine the alkaline food list and see what to be consumed now.

Foods on that are alkaline-producing are veggies, seeds, the majority of fruits, brown rice and other grains, and fish. These foods can be combined and matched to your own choice for a minimum of 80% of your total diet plan, and then you add 20% of the acidic-producing foods, and the acidic foods are not all "bad." Foods on the acidic side are entire grain bread, lean meats, milk and milk products, butter and eggs, and this includes up to make a 100% alkaline diet.

To monitor your pH level as soon as you have started on an alkaline diet plan and cancer combating method of eating, check any natural food shop for pH strips or litmus paper. There will be a color chart included to utilize and determine what your pH blood level is. For an alkaline system, it should register between 7.2 - 7.8. No 2 individuals are alike, so check your pH level about when a day as you get going. Continue to inspect when a week. Eat more alkaline foods and use green supplements if you require to raise your pH level. An alkaline diet plan will prevent illness naturally.

# An ALKALINE DIET FOR HEALTH AND WEIGHT LOSS

There is a lot of insane diets on the market that pledge to help you slim down. If you look at the dietary worth of some of these diets, they are often badly lacking. If you require to slim down, you must do it while consuming a diet that is excellent for your body, so you will turn out to be a lot more beneficial rather than essentially more slender. An alkaline diet is a sound way to deal with weight decrease that will keep you stimulated, healthy, and encouraged to drop the pounds.

## Comprehending the Alkaline Diet

An alkaline diet is not quite the same as different diets, because of the way that it centers principally around the effect that nourishments have on the causticity or the alkalinity of the body. At the point when nourishments are processed and utilized by the body, they produce what much of the time portrayed as an "alkaline debris" or "corrosive debris is."The original pH of the food does not factor into this last result within the body. In truth, a couple of the most acidic nourishments, for example, natural citrusproducts, really produce an alkaline outcome when eaten. At the point when progressively alkaline nourishments are eaten rather than corrosive nourishments, the pH of the body can be changed to an ideal degree of around 7.3. While this isn't amazingly alkaline, it is sufficient to pick up bunches of stimulating preferences.

## Utilizing an Alkaline Diet for Weight Loss

Many individuals attempt fad diet plans or those who promise fast lead to an effort to drop weight. These diets might produce lead to the short-term; however, with time, this can be an extremely unhealthy way to slim down. Additionally, many individuals gain the weight back as quickly as they go off their rigorous diet plan. When an acid diet plan is used for weight reduction and control, it is more of a lifestyle change. The outcomes may not happen overnight, but it's most likely that the weight will not be gained back. An alkaline diet plan is rich in foods that are naturally low in calories, such as the majority of fruits and vegetables. Much of the foods that are high in fat and calories are also acidifying, so when these foods are eliminated from the diet, a natural and healthy weight-loss will occur. These foods consist of red meat, fatty foods, high fat dairy products such as whole milk and cheese, soda, sugar, and alcohol. As soon as you stop consuming these foods, your body will be much healthier, less acid, and you'll likewise drop weight while doing so. Due to the fact that the diet is healthy, you can stay with it long term. Many people who begin an alkaline diet entirely for the purpose of losing weight find numerous other advantages. An increased energy level, resistance to illness, and an overall enhancement in health and well-being are amongst the numerous advantages you can experience on an alkaline diet.

## How to Start an Alkaline Diet

Lots of people discover that it is much easier to start on an alkaline diet plan by making small changes. Start by gradually reducing the amount of meat, sugar and fat in your diet plan while including fresh fruits, vegetables, healthy fats such as olive oil, almonds, soy products, and natural sweeteners such as Stevia. You'll find gradually, your tastes will change, and you'll really begin to choose this type of diet.

# ALKALINE DIET - HOW DOES IT HELP?

Alkaline Diet, also referred to as Alkaline Acid Diet, is a diet based upon usage of food such as fruits, veggies, nuts, roots, and vegetables however prevent dairy, meat, salts and grains. Just recently, this diet has gained appeal among diet and nutrition professionals and authors. It is still in dispute with the performance of an alkaline diet because there is no concrete evidence that an alkaline diet can lower particular diseases.

As aforementioned, fruits, veggies, vegetables, roots, and nuts are part of the alkaline diet plan. The alkaline diet plan refers to the diet plan of having more of alkaline-producing food.

## Alkaline Diet

Our blood has a pH between 7.35 and 7.45, which is a little alkaline. The alkaline diet is based on this pH level of our blood and any diet that is high in acid-producing food will disorganise the balance. When the body attempts to renew the stability of pH in the blood, the acidity of the food will contribute to the loss of essential minerals such as potassium, salt, calcium, and magnesium. The imbalance will make people prone to disease.

Western diets are more acid-producing and they consume little fresh fruits and veggies. Due to the development of an alkaline diet, the standard of the Western diet plan has actually altered considerably.

Some diet and nutrition professionals think that acid-producing diet plan may cause some persistent health problem and following signs such as:

- headache
- sluggish
- regular influenza and cold, and excess mucous production
- anxiety, uneasiness
- polycystic ovaries, ovarian cysts, benign breast cysts

Some think the above conditions are the result of acid-producing diet plan, and usage of vegetables and fruits is advantageous to health, some physicians believe that acid-producing diet plan does not trigger persistent illness. Besides that, there is evidence shown that alkaline diets assist in preventing the development of calcium kidney stones, osteoporosis, and age-related muscle wasting.

## Balance diet plan

The alkaline diet is preferred; it is not recommended to have a severe diet (consume all alkaline-producing food). It is healthier to strive for a balanced, happy medium of both kinds of food. Simply keep in mind to keep in mind the tips above and speak with a practitioner/doctor before you desire to try a brand-new diet plan.

# THE PERKS OF THE ALKALINE DIET PROGRAM

Some diet plans put constraints on what foods can be eaten due to the fact that of what's in them, while others are laxer with food selection; however, strict on when you can consume. The alkaline diet can be classified into the latter, as it consists of taking in healthy foods, however, can eventually result in weight loss.

The pH level of the human body is expected to be around 7.35, which is slightly alkaline and indicates that alkaline is needed by the body. Hunters and collectors ages back had no problem meeting this requirement as the majority of the foods they are were abundant in alkalines, such as nuts, vegetables, and seeds.

Nowadays, nevertheless, the contemporary day diet is not extremely alkaline, consisting primarily of processed foods and animal protein. When these foods and other products such as coffee, beans, and fish are taken in, they release acids that happen to compromise our bones.

The alkaline diet plan is appealing because it promotes strength in the bones and joints. Acid weakens the bones, so consuming a diet high in alkaline will offset the effects that acids have on our bodies.

Extra advantages of the alkaline diet consist of increased energy levels and decreasing excess mucous production. It can likewise assist those who struggle with influenza, colds, and nasal blockage regularly. Likewise, those who have other symptoms such as polycystic ovaries, ovarian cysts, and benign breast cysts can enhance by changing to an alkaline based diet plan. Finally, it can minimize feelings of anxiousness, irritability, and stress and anxiety.

# HEALTH BENEFITS OF AN ALKALINE DIET

The Many Health Benefits of an Alkaline Diet
There are numerous reasons an individual might choose to go on an alkaline diet plan. Due to the fact that it has numerous healthful benefits, it is typical for a person to go on a diet for one particular factor, only to find lots of other enhancements in their life as a result. Here are some of the health advantages of an alkaline diet that might make it the right choice for you:

## Improved Energy Levels

An alkaline diet is understood for the boost it can provide to a person's energy level. The typical diet is high in processed grains, processed sugar, food, and fat additives which can drain a person's energy level. It's simpler for your body to digest these natural foods, so you won't experience that dip in your energy level after consuming, which is so typical with a fatty and sugary diet.

## Resistance to Disease and Illness

An alkaline diet is also the very best choice if you wish to help to minimize your possibilities of getting ill. The body is much better geared up to combat disease if it is not likewise encumbered the effects of level of acidity. When your body's pH is kept at an approximate level of 7.3, all bodily functions will be able to work at peak efficiency, including your coronary, respiratory, and gastrointestinal systems. As an included bonus, the foods that are frequently eaten as part of an alkaline diet plan are natural, fresh and healthy. Processed foods, the majority of which are acidifying, contain food ingredients and chemicals that can really contribute to the toxicity of the body. When your body is fighting toxicity, it is more prone to disease. By removing these foods from your diet, you'll increase your total health level. A high acid level in the body can likewise encourage the development of particular diseases, such as cancer. By keeping your body's pH at a slightly alkaline level, you'll be making it more resistant to the development of these diseases. Numerous people also discover an increased resistance to allergies and fewer breathing problems when they change to an alkaline diet plan. This is typically due to the fact that numerous acid producing foods are likewise mucous producing foods. When these foods are eliminated from the diet, nasal and lung blockage is reduced and much better breathing can take place.

## Weight Loss and Weight Control

An alkaline diet plan is likewise a wonderful option for weight-loss and weight control. The majority of alkaline foods are high in nutrients and yet low in calories and fat. When you switch to an alkaline diet plan, you'll be providing your body the optimal nutrition it needs, while reducing your caloric consumption. The gastrointestinal system can likewise function more effectively on an alkaline diet plan, so you'll be getting more nutrition from the foods you consume, even at lower calorie levels.

# QUICK AND EASY ALKALINE DIET SHORTCUTS

An alkaline diet plan can be one of the very best methods of increasing your overall health and sense of well-being. Some individuals incorrectly think that "eating alkaline" is made complex and difficult to do, it's actually extremely simple to switch your diet plan from one that is excessively acid to one that is healthy and alkaline. There are some fast and simple ways to get fast outcomes if you desire to experience lots of health advantages of an alkaline diet plan. You can experience better health, better disease resistance, and an increased level of energy, to name a few benefits, merely from changing to an alkaline diet plan.

## Include Alkaline Water to Your Diet

Drinking plenty of water is vital to excellent health, so why not make the many of it by drinking alkaline water? For a tasty and alkalizing beverage, include a squeeze of fresh lemon to your alkaline water prior to drinking. You can likewise utilize it to make healthy organic and green teas, both of which are alkaline drinks.

## Consume Plenty of Salads

Salads made from lettuce, spinach, and other leafy green vegetables are fantastic alkaline diet plan additions. By merely including a fresh tossed salad to your lunch and dinner menu, you'll be improving your health in addition to alkalizing your body. Nearly all veggies are alkalizing, so you'll have lots of options to keep your salads amazing and intriguing. Try adding chopped cucumbers, snow peas, fresh green peas, and green pepper strips to your salad. You can even add a bit of protein by consisting of beans and other beans.

## Consume Less Sugar

Refined sugar is very damaging to one's health, especially because it motivates an acidic reaction within the body. You can also change white processed sugar with a bit of raw sugar, maple sugar, or Stevia, which are all alkalizing sweetening options.

## Easy Food Substitutions

It's simple to change your diet from being extremely acidifying to alkalizing by simply making a couple of basic food replacements. Rather than processed noodles and pasta, eat entire grains such as millet, quinoa and wild rice. Replace the red meat in your diet plan with fish, beans and other vegetables for protein. Use healthy fats in your foods, such as olive, flax seed, or canola oil. You must likewise eat a diet plan that is abundant in fresh vegetables and fruits because many are alkalizing. Before you know it, you'll be feeling much better and reaping the health benefits of an alkaline diet.
ALKALINE DIET - HOW IT WORKS
The alkaline diet is actually simply the reverse of high fat, high protein, low carbohydrate diet that has actually ended up being the standard in current years. Yet it could benefit you if you haven't heard of an alkaline diet plan. You aren't alone.

If you feel inadequate if you consume a diet plan low in carbs and high in protein, you must think about the alkaline diet. If you have symptoms of the excess level of acidity, you should also consider it. These signs include persistent fatigue, low energy, nasal congestion, frequent infections or colds, anxious, nervous, stressed, dry hair and/or skin, weak nails, muscle discomfort, leg cramps, hives, and gastritis.

Prior to you start, you can measure your salivary pH and see what it is. This is an acidic result if its extremely low such as a 4. If it's high such as an 8, then this is alkaline. Once you understand what your pH is and you know which foods are alkaline and which are acidic, you can begin to balance things and return and keep your body at an alkaline pH.

There are numerous charts available online free of charge that can provide the information. Let's look at few alkaline fruits - bananas, apples, coconut, nectarines, pineapple, and tomatoes are simply a couple of. Alfalfa, celery, cabbage, carrots, garlic, lettuce, and mushrooms are a few of the alkaline vegetables. There are likewise alkaline dairy cereals, nuts, and products.

How does it work? A lot of foods are either alkaline or acidic depending upon the residue they leave in the body and how they are metabolized. It's an excellent idea to pursue a balance in the body with simply a slight alkalinity. You must not assume your diet is too acidic or to alkaline based on what you eat. There are many things that can impact the pH of the body. For example, an orange is acidic when you consume it but turns alkaline in the body.

An alkaline diet that keeps the body somewhat alkaline can benefit you by improving your overall health. There is speculation that it might avoid cancer cells from establishing, and an alkaline diet has shown to make some chemo drugs more powerful and more reliable.

Although there might not be a good deal of direct research study on the alkaline diet plan, there is a lot of research that reveals that individuals who are sick most times have acidic blood, which leads to an imbalance. Hardly ever is blood too alkaline, so you do not need to worry about consuming a lot of alkaline foods.

Here are a couple of sample dishes.
- Green Raw Soup
- 2 Avocados
- 1 Cucumber, peel, and seed
- 1 Jalapeno pepper, seeded
- 1 Yellow or red onion, diced
- Juice of 1/2 Lemon
- 1-2 cups Water or Veggie stock
- 2 cloves roasted Garlic
- 1 Tbsp. Coriander
- 1 Tbsp. Parsley

Steps:
Puree all components (except onions) in a food processor or mixer. Add basically water to desired
consistency. Leading with diced onions for garnish.

Autumn Tomato & Avocado Soup
Ingredients:
- 5 big ripe tomatoes.
- 2 ripe avocados
- 1/2 spring onion
- 1/4 cup ground almonds
- 1 cup broth from a natural vegetable stock without any preservatives or artificial additives
- 1/4 teaspoon dill seed
- Dash cayenne pepper

- Sea salt & split black pepper to taste

Directions:
Just simply put all of the ingredients into a blender and mix!
Location the soup into a pan and warm.

The alkaline diet might not be for everyone but is certainly the right choice for some. If you think that the Alkaline diet plan might assist you, talk to your doctor prior to you begin it.

# THE ALKALINE DIET - WHAT CAN I EAT ON IT?

Putting together an effective alkaline diet needs taking in the correct foods and in the correct amounts. Your alkaline diet plan menu is crucial to diets' success. In this book, you will discover why alkaline diet plans are helpful to our health, how you can successfully implement your diet, and which foods you must put on your alkaline diet plan menu.

## The History of Human Diet

Early man's diet plan was far various from what we consume today. A run of the mill human diet today comprises of significantly more creature proteins. Extreme salts, phony sugars, and additives increase the acidity of our current diet plans.

How Alkaline Diets Work

By purposely managing the acid to alkaline balance in your body, you are able to gain from a vast array of health advantages. Increased energy and weight-loss will be immediately obvious to somebody who is recently going back to stabilize from an extremely acidic body. By making your diet plan out of around 75% alkaline nourishments and just 25% acidic food sources, you can restore your body to its sound, regular state. Additionally, setting up the acidic nourishments with alkaline water can extraordinarily diminish their acidifying influence on the body.An alkaline diet works to minimize the tension put on your liver, kidneys, and other organs by having an extremely acidic (poisonous) body.

## Your Alkaline Diet Menu

The following are arrangements of various nourishments which are our top proposals for having an alkaline diet. While nourishments that are acidic ought to be ingested for a solid diet, they are too be brought down to the levels which our bodies at first adjusted to.

Alkaline Fruits:

- apples
- bananas
- blackberries
- dates
- oranges
- pineapple
- raisins

Alkaline Vegetables:

- broccoli
- cabbage
- carrots
- cauliflower
- celery
- eggplant
- mushrooms
- squash
- turnips

Acidic foods should make up no more than 25% of your diet plan. Noted below are the types of food which are acidic. Remember that every category listed below has foods that are badly acidic, however likewise some which are much more on the alkaline side.

Acidic Foods:
- meat
- cheese
- vegetables
- grains
- nuts
- select fruits
- select vegetables

# 14-DAY MEAL PLAN

Diabetic patients must never skip meals or snacks and must eat at the same fixed schedule every day. Using an exchange list can be helpful in maintaining variety in food intake while ensuring the appropriate mix of carbohydrates, proteins, calories, and other food nutrients. In this way, dieting does not turn into a struggle. By using an exchange list, persons with diabetes will find it easier to make wise choices with their food intake.

There is no standard or fixed diabetic diet plan. All eating plans should be flexible and should consider the lifestyle and the specific health needs of each patient. Aside from keeping glucose levels within moderate range, a diabetic diet is also meant to reduce the risk for the complications that may result from diabetes such as cardiovascular diseases, hypertension or renal failure. A good diet can lessen the other risk factors that may further aggravate the diabetic condition such as obesity, hypertension, and bad cholesterol.

## Less Fat, More Fruits and Vegetables

Seeking the professional help of a registered dietitian can also be helpful. A dietitian can help a diabetes patient develop a meal plan that would tell what kind of food can be best eaten during meals and the amounts needed to keep body glucose within normal levels. In most diabetic patients, a healthy meal plan consists of 20% to 60% of calories from carbohydrates, 20% for protein, and 30% or preferably less from fat.

Generally, at every meal, a diabetic person may have two to five choices of carbohydrates or up to 60 grams, 1 choice of protein, and a small amount of fat. Carbohydrates are best when derived from fruits, vegetables, dairy, and starchy foods. Diabetic patients should also avoid preserved food. Fresh fruits and vegetables are especially good for diabetics.

# Poultry and Fish for Protein

On the other hand, protein can be taken from meat, poultry or fish. Poultry and fish should be preferred than red meat like pork or beef. Extra fat and poultry skin should be avoided. Finally, fat can be found in products such as butter, margarine, lard, and oil. It can also be derived from dairy and meat. Diabetics, as much as possible, should avoid fried foods, egg yolks, bacon, and other high-fat products.

Caution should also be observed in consuming processed food products. Before eating any of processed food products, a diabetic patient should look at the "nutrition facts" label on the packaging. In this way, one is able to determine what kind of processed food products are healthy and what are to be avoided.

If a diabetic patient closely follows one's diet plan - eating the right kind of food, ensuring the right serving sizes, and sticking to the fixed meal schedule - one will be assured of consuming a consistent amount of carbohydrates, calories, proteins, and fats every day. Without a diet plan, it becomes difficult for a diabetic patient to control glucose levels in the blood. Uncontrolled high glucose levels can increase risks of further diabetic complications.

Being creative within the rules of a diabetic diet plan can also help maintain variety in food preferences makes eating as healthy and normal as other people. With good food and a good free diabetic diet plan, even persons with diabetes can look forward to a good and healthy life ahead.

The kidney diet (renal diet) can be one of the most challenging aspects of living with chronic kidney disease. Not only do you need to determine, with the help of a dietitian, what foods are good (and bad) for you, but then come up with meals that are satisfying and enjoyable as well.We've compiled a collection of recipes that we find are tasty, but also kidney-friendly.At the bottom of each recipe you will find nutritional guidelines to help you stay in line with your personal needs. Every person is different and each meal may need adjusting depending on your situation, so please be sure to check with your dietitian or medical team if you're not sure about a recipe.

# DAY 1

## MEXICAN EGG & TORTILLA SKILLET

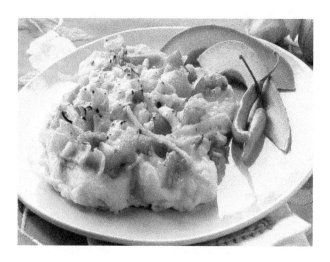

### Ingredients

8 eggs (or egg beaters)
2 green onions, sliced thin, with some green showing
1 teaspoon chili powder
1/4 cup low salt ketchup
2 Tablespoon Butter
1 bag (6oz) unsalted tortilla chips*, broken up

### Direction

Beat eggs until well blended.
Add the onion, chili powder, and ketchup. Beat again until well mixed. Set aside.
Melt butter in a skillet, then add the tortilla chips and sauté over moderate heat until warmed through. Stir in egg mixture and scramble until the desired consistency.Serve at once on heated plates.
*If you cannot find unsalted tortilla chips then you can take flour tortillas and cut in fourths. Bake at 350°F until crisp.

# DAY 2

## FRESH FRUIT

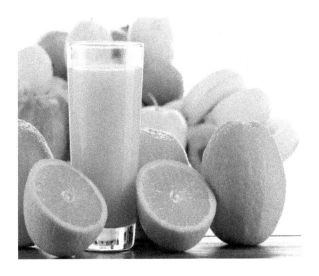

**Delicious and refreshing and renal-friendly any time of the year**

Makes 8 portions
Serving Size 1/2 cup

## Ingredients

1/2 cup Strawberries, fresh or frozen
1/2 cup Blackberries, fresh or frozen
1/2 cup Blueberries, fresh or frozen
1/2 cup Peaches, pared, cut
1/4 cup Red raspberries, fresh or frozen, sweetened, not thawed
1/2 cup Orange juice, fresh or canned, unsweetened
1 Apple, cut into bite-size pieces
1 Banana, cut into bite size pieces

## Directions

Pour orange juice into a large container.
Add all ingredients listed.
Toss gently.
When using frozen fruit, allow 4 hours at room temperature for thawing

# DAY 3

## BURRITOS WITH EGGS AND MEXICAN SAUSAGE

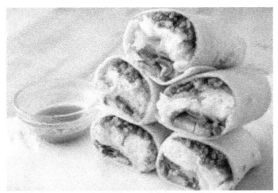

Delicious and filling, kidney friendly breakfast for any day of the week and for on the go. Wrap it up and take it with you!
Servings: 3

## Ingredients

3 ounces of chorizo (Mexican sausage)
3 eggs, beaten
3 flour tortillas

## Directions

1.  Fry chorizo in skillet until dark in color.
2.  Add eggs and cook until done.
3.  Fill warmed tortillas with mixture and roll up, folding up the bottom edge before rolling to keep the filling from falling out.

# DAY 4

## ORANGE FLAVORED COFFEE

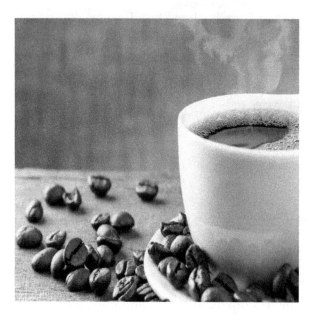

Treat your holiday guests (and yourself) to something special after dinner with our orange flavored coffee recipe.
Servings: 20
Serving Size: 2 round teaspoons

### Ingredients

1/2 cup instant coffee
3/4 cup sugar
1 cup Coffee Mate Powder
1/2 teaspoon dried orange peel

**Directions**

1. Blend the above ingredients in a blender until powdered.
2. For each serving, place 2 round teaspoons of coffee mix in a cup and add
boiling water.

# DAY 5

## LOW SALT MACARONI AND CHEESE

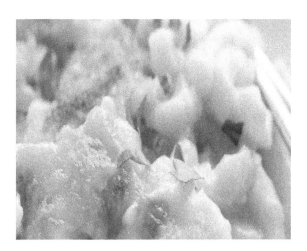

Everyone's favorite comfort food is just as delicious without all the sodium. This low salt macaroni and cheese recipe will satisfy the whole family!
Servings: 4

## Ingredients

2 cups noodles, (any shape you want)
2 to 3 cups boiling water
1/2 cup grated cheddar cheese
1 teaspoon margarine or salt free butter
1/4 teaspoon dried mustard

## Directions

1. Boil water, add noodles, cook about 5-7 minutes till tender.
2. Drain.
3. While still very hot, sprinkle with cheese, stir in butter and mustard.
(Optional – Bake at 350 for ten to fifteen minutes or until top is golden brown for an extra yummy crunch.)
Chicken Salad
Servings: 4
Dressing
1/2 cup olive oil
1/4 cup vinegar
1/2 teaspoon white pepper
1/4 teaspoon basil
1 teaspoon sugar
Salad
3 cups cooked fusilli pasta (any pasta shape will work)
8 ounces cold cooked chicken, diced
1/2 cup frozen peas, defrosted
1/2cup chopped red pepper
1 cup sliced zucchini
1 medium carrot, sliced thinly
2 cups shredded lettuce

## Directions

1. Put dressing ingredients in jar with lid and shake to blend ingredients. Chill for at least 2 hours. Shake again before mixing with salad.
2. Mix together pasta, chicken, peas, zucchini, red pepper and carrot in large bowl.
3. Add dressing and toss well. Divide lettuce onto 4 plates and top with salad mixture.

Italian Eggplant Salad

Servings; 4

Ingredients

3 cups cubed eggplant
1 small onion, chopped
2 tablespoons white wine vinegar
1 clove garlic, chopped
1/2 teaspoon oregano
1/4 teaspoon black pepper
1 medium tomato, chopped
3 tablespoons olive oil

## Directions

1. Add eggplant to boiling water in saucepan.
2. Reheat to boiling; reduce heat.
3. Cover and cook until tender, about 10 minutes; drain.
4. Place eggplant and onion in glass dish.
5. Mix together vinegar, garlic, and pepper.
6. Pour over eggplant and onion; toss.
7. Stir in oil just before serving.

# DAY 6

## HAWAIIAN CHICKEN SALAD

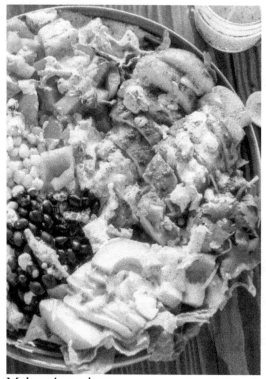

Makes 4 servings
Serving Size: 3/4 cup

### Ingredients

1/2 Cup Diced Celery
1-1/4 Cups Shredded Head of Lettuce
1-1/2 Cups Chopped Cooked Chicken
1 Cup Drained Unsweetened Pineapple Chunks

1/2 tsp. Sugar
2 tsp. Lemon Juice
1/2 Cup Mayonnaise
Dash Tabasco Sauce
1/4 tsp. Pepper
Paprika

## Directions

1. Place celery, lettuce, chicken, and pineapple in a bowl.
2. Mix sugar, lemon juice, mayonnaise, Tabasco, and pepper together.
3. Add to chicken mixture and toss to mix.
4. Serve on a lettuce leaf and sprinkle with paprika.

# DAY 7

## CHICKEN WALDORF SALAD

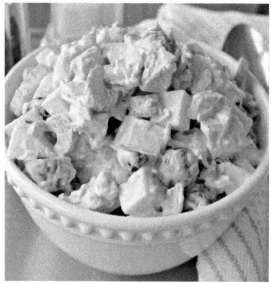

Servings: 4
Serving Size: About 3/4 cup

### Ingredients

8 ounces chicken or turkey, cooked and cubed
1/2 cup apple, chopped
1/2 cup celery, chopped
2 tablespoons raisins
1/2 tablespoon ground ginger (optional)
1/2 cup Miracle Whip

## Directions

1. Mix together until well blended.
2. It is best if it can sit in the fridge for a while to blend flavors.

# DAY 8

## CHICKEN AND BOW-TIE PASTA

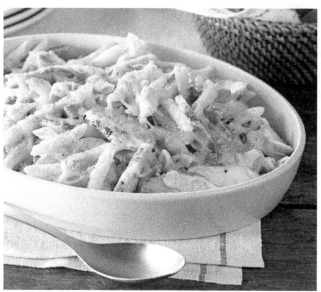

Servings: 6

### Ingredients

3 cups cooked bow-tie pasta (any shape will work)
8 ounces chicken breast
2 cloves garlic
1/4 cup olive oil
1-1/2 cups chopped broccoli (frozen)
1/2 cup chopped green onions
1 cup chopped red pepper
1 teaspoon ground basil
1/4 teaspoon cayenne pepper

3/4 cup white wine
1 cup low sodium chicken broth (or homemade without salt)
Directions
1. Sauté garlic in oil in large skillet.
2. Add chicken breast cut into small strips and brown.
3. Add remaining ingredients and simmer for 15 minutes.
4. Toss with cooked bow-tie pasta and serve immediately.

# DAY 9

## BURRITOS RAPIDOS

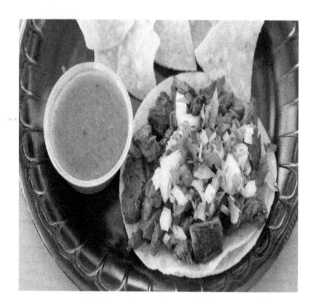

This juicy, flavorful and kidney friendly fajitas recipe proves that sticking to your renal diet plan doesn't doesn't have to be bland and boring. Make it extra fun and bring the sizzling skillet to the table to serve it Mexican restaurant style.
Servings: 4

### Ingredients

4  Corn tortillas (much lower in sodium than wheat)
1/2 cup diced red or green pepper
1/2 cup diced green or white onion
2  eggs or leftover meat, fish or chicken

Toppings:
grated cheddar cheese, sour cream, lettuce, fresh salsa (See Sixty-Second Salsa recipe in the "Side Dishes," category.)
Directions
1. Spray fry pan with non-stick spray. Add peppers and onion and cook until onion is translucent, and peppers are bright in color.
2. Add eggs or meat and cook, stirring occasionally, until done.
3. Meanwhile, wrap corn tortillas in wet paper towel, microwave for 1 minute or so.
4. Serve with toppings.

# DAY 10

## CAULIFLOWER IN MUSTARD SAUCE

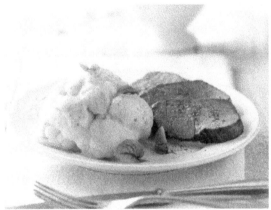

Servings: 4

### Ingredients

2 teaspoons Dijon mustard
1 teaspoon honey
1 tablespoon + 2 teaspoons white-wine vinegar
1 tablespoon olive oil
Dash black pepper

2 cups cauliflower flowerettes

## Directions

1. Whisk together the mustard and honey; whisk in the vinegar and then the olive oil.
2. Season with some black pepper. Set aside.
3. Add the cauliflower to boiling water and cook until tender.
4. Drain well.
5. Toss the drained, cooked cauliflower with the dressing.
6. Allow to cool for 30-45 minutes and serve.

# DAY 11

## PINEAPPLE CREAM CAKE

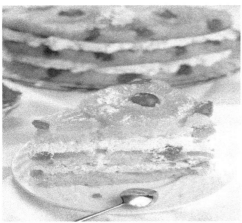

Serve this pineapple cream cake for breakfast or an after dinner dessert.
Servings: 18

### Ingredients

1 8-oz pkg.cream cheese, softened
1/4 cup sugar
5 large eggs
1 8-oz can crushed pineapple, drained
1 box yellow cake mix (about 18 ounces)
1/3 cup vegetable oil
1 cup water
1    teaspoon vanilla flavoring
Directions

1. Preheat the oven to the temperature recommended on the box of cake mix.

2. In a small bowl, combine cream cheese, sugar, and two eggs, beating well. Stir in

Drained pineapple and set aside.

3. In a large bowl, combine the yellow cake mix, oil, water, vanilla flavoring, and

remaining three eggs. Beat with an electric mixer at high speed for two minutes.

4. Spray either a Bundt pan or a 9 X 3.5-inch tube pan with cooking spray and cover

with flour.

5. Add the cream cheese mixture to the cake batter, mixing well. Then pour the batter

into the greased and floured pan.

6. Bake for 55 to 65 minutes or until the center is set. Test for doneness by inserting a

butter knife into the center of the cake. Cool in the pan for 10 minutes.

# DAY 12

## APPLE PANCAKE

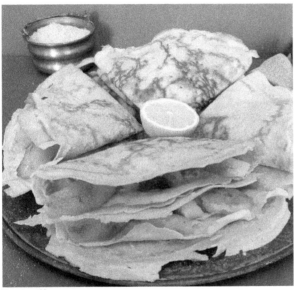

Ingredients
2 tablespoons unsalted butter
3 large Granny Smith apples, peeled and sliced
6 tablespoons granulated sugar
1 teaspoon ground cinnamon
3 eggs
1/2 cup all-purpose flour
1/2 cup milk
1 tablespoon sour cream
1/4 teaspoon salt
1 teaspoon grated lemon zest
Instructions
1. Melt butter over medium-high heat in an ovenproof pan.
2. Add apples, sugar and cinnamon; sauté and stir 3-5 minutes. Remove from

heat.

3. In a bowl, beat eggs until frothy. Add flour, milk, sour cream, salt and zest.

Beat until smooth batter forms.

4. Pour over apples and bake in 400 F degree oven until puffed and golden

brown, about 25 minutes.

5. Cut into wedge and serve directly from the pan.

Optional: drizzle honey or dust with powdered sugar.

# DAY 13

## SPICY PORK CHOPS

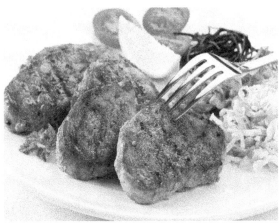

Try these Spicy Pork Chops with apple and onion for a tasty, family meal.

Makes 6 servings.

2 Garlic cloves, pared, minced

3/4 tsp. Salt

1.2 tsp. Ground ginger

1/2 tsp. Sugar

1/4 tsp. Pepper

1/4 tsp. Ground cumin

6 large pork chops

2 Medium Rome Beauty apples, unpared, cored, cut into 1-in slices

1 Large red onion, pared, cut into 3/4-in slices

1. Combine first six ingredients.
2. Rub seasoning mixture into both sides of each pork chop.
3. Place in large glass pan.
4. Insert slices of apples and onions between chops.

5. Crumple aluminum foil and place at each end of pan to press ingredients together.
6. Cover with foil; bake at 400F for 20 minutes.
7. Reduce heat to 325F; bake for 30 to 35 minutes.
8. Uncover.
9. Remove crumpled foil to separate chops; bake for about 15 minutes until light brown.
10. Serve over rice.
Serving size 1 chop.
Calories 215 kcal
Protein 15 gm
Fat 13 gm
Carbohydrate 9.8 gm
Cholesterol 52 mg
Sodium 330 mg
Potassium 288 mg
Phosphorus 126 mg

# DAY 14

## LOW SODIUM POUND CAKE

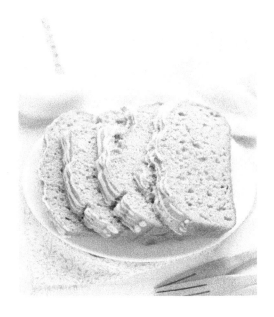

### Ingredients

1/4 lb Butter, unsalted
3/4 cup Sugar
2 large eggs, beaten slightly
1 1/4 cup Bread flour
3 oz. Milk

## Directions

Cream butter and gradually add sugar.
Beat until fluffy.
Add eggs, flour and milk.
Mix well.
Line 18×13 in pan with pan paper.
Bake at 375 F for 30 minutes.

Nutritional Value
Calories 243
Protein 3.7 g
Fat 12 g
Carbohydrate 31 g
Fiber .6 g
Cholesterol 75 mg
Sodium 18 mg
Potassium 47 mg
Phosphorus 45 mg

CPSIA information can be obtained
at www.ICGtesting.com
Printed in the USA
BVHW062330010321
601388BV00009B/1213